Table of Contents

5.2. Technological Advancements

The Role of Biomarkers in Diagnosing Alzheimer's Disease

1. Introduction to Alzheimer's Disease

Since both PET and CSF diagnostics are still expensive and invasive or poorly available in subspecialty medical centers on an international basis, ability to reach the AD diagnosis at lower-cost, noninvasive and wider entrees is dependent on the further discovery of more sensitive and more special biomarkers or biomarker combinations in the blood. Such biomarker assays could also aid the physicians in tracking or monitoring, in some occasions in seeking precision in the treatment of certainly undiagnosed AD or other dementia disorders. Different biomarker tools can detect different neuronal injury and apoptosis, tissue malformation, cell speed of progression, or their associations or interactions.

Alzheimer's disease (AD) is the most prevalent cause of dementia around the world. This neurodegenerative disorder is associated with increased age and usually starts with memory loss and has further symptoms, such as decline in other cognitive domains, psychiatric and behavioral disorders, and functional impairment. Currently, neuropathologic diagnosis after death is the most sufficient or 'golden standard' instrument for the definite diagnosis of AD. Neuropathologic hallmarks include several intertwined or twisted structures and clumps: amyloid-β plaques, tau neurofibrillary tangles, degenerated neurons, and synapses. Biomarkers can be short for 'biological markers', which can be measured as reliable signs or indicators for biological states or

conditions modern techniques. These foretell the
probability, risk, and behavior of certain disease processes,
such as AD.

1.1. Definition and Prevalence

Biochemical changes take place in the brains of people with Alzheimer's Disease, like reduced levels of neurotransmitters such as acetylcholine in particular regions of the brain and increased amounts of amyloid protein, tau, or both kinds in the spaces affected. The quantity of acetylcholine present is not a direct cause for reduced memory or mood variations, nor does the presence of amyloid plaques and neurofibrillary tangles appear to lead to dementia. Even considering this information, the presence of amyloid plaques and tangles in the brain is still a hallmark of Alzheimer's Disease. Quantifying these measures and combining information about these proteins with known symptoms, imaging results, and other available information can lead to more accurate conclusions made concerning the probable diagnosis of the disease.

The National Institute on Aging defines Alzheimer's Disease as "an irreversible, progressive brain disorder that slowly destroys memory and thinking skills and, eventually, the ability to carry out the simplest tasks." While the majority of those with the condition are over the age of 65, early onset of the disease is also observed in individuals. Though statistics are approximate, it is known that the number of individuals diagnosed with Alzheimer's Disease is definitely growing; those over the age of 65 are most likely to be diagnosed, with a 3% chance in people between the ages of 65 and 74. The likelihood of a person getting Alzheimer's Disease increases through age, rising from 10% - 30% in those 85 or older. In fact, the average span of time an individual survives after a diagnosis is 3 or 4 years, but those capable of living up to 20 years past diagnosis often spend a majority of their time being cared for by others because of their diminished physical and mental capacities.

1.2. Symptoms and Progression

At the symptomatic stage, Alzheimer's disease (AD) is characterized by the presence of β-amyloid and tau in the brain. Biomarkers for β-amyloid and tau have been recognized and are of great use for both the diagnosis and prognosis of AD. Several brain imaging techniques have been developed for AD, such as computerized tomography (CT), magnetic resonance imaging (MRI), and positron emission tomography (PET). Although numerous promising results have been presented in the context of AD for these imaging techniques, after the bronchoscope (CSF) investigation, it is troublesome for people with mild cognitive impairment. Between the CSF techniques, sub-cognitive impairment, and biomarkers imaging, many studies have found considerable variation in subjects, but there are only a few reports to incorporate all three stage biomarkers into a single diagnostic test.

Alzheimer's disease is a degenerative disorder that occurs when a protein fragment known as beta-amyloid clumps together to form amyloid plaques. As more beta-amyloid is produced and spreads, a toxic heap of dead nerve cells and protein is flanked with tangles of another type of protein called tau, which blocks internal transport. AD takes about 10 to 20 years between the onset of abnormalities and the emergence of clinical symptoms.

Alzheimer's is typically characterized by two main types of protein clumps in and around brain cells. Using biomarkers is an early indicator of Alzheimer's pathology.

2. Understanding Biomarkers

There are many biomarkers for Alzheimer's Disease diagnosis and can be divided into two categories: dementia biomarkers and AD-specific biomarkers. Dementia biomarkers could help clinicians understand brain ß-amyloid and Tau pathophysiology, calculated using positive and negative of amyloid and tau in CSF PET. The top several biomarkers for Alzheimer's Disease are also amyloid beta and different total tau levels. Amanda Hawkins et al. also revealed that ß-amyloid, CSF Tau level, and brain atrophy using MRI AD-signature predicted Alzheimer's Disease dementia. Another study discussed their biomarkers prediction, like the amyloid positron emission tomography predicted Alzheimer's Disease or MRI semi-quantitative score of 2.5 and 0.33 of CSF AD signature gave the maximal accuracy of AD classification.

Biomarkers are characteristics that can be objectively measured and evaluated as indicators of biological processes. In the context of Alzheimer's Disease, a biomarker may be a change in amyloid or tau in the cerebrospinal fluid (CSF) or the presence of a specific kind of brain atrophy visible on a magnetic resonance imaging (MRI) brain scan. Biomarkers surrounding the brain can be costly and require hospital infrastructure and specialized expertise to measure. There are blood, cerebrospinal fluid (CSF), and imaging (PET & MRI) biomarkers. There is no "silver bullet" biomarker for Alzheimer's Disease diagnosis that can provide an accurate conclusion. However, using

various types of tests to confirm the result can lead to a
more accurate diagnosis.

2.1. Definition and Types of Biomarkers

Central nervous system changes correlated with the development of abnormal protein aggregates in amyloid plaques and neurofibrillary tangles consist of another hallmark of AD. Therefore, using cerebrospinal fluid and neuroimaging to detect amyloid-beta is a promising approach. In consensus criteria, cerebrospinal fluid and amyloid imaging abnormalities related to brain accumulation of beta-amyloid have defined an AD predictive biomarker signature. As the amyloid biomarker first appears to be consistent with the clinical symptoms, amyloid biomarkers are associated with AD diagnosis. As part of the research diagnostic guidelines, another consistent diagnostic biomarker is magnetic resonance imaging measures of neurodegeneration.

Biomarkers are biological measurements that serve to help predict the clinical course of a target disorder, and there are several types, including risk factor biomarkers, detectable disease biomarkers, monitoring of disease activity biomarkers, and prognosis and/or treatment outcome biomarkers. Risk factor biomarkers measure the probabilities of developing symptoms and perform different supplementary functions, among which genetics and plasma amyloid are used for diagnosing Alzheimer's Disease (AD). For detectable disease biomarkers, it can determine the likelihood of ever displaying signs and symptoms of target disorders and thus diagnostic tools using in vivo imaging were developed. Meanwhile, monitoring of disease activity biomarkers is established using systems biology and supports interpreting clinical symptoms, while prognosis and/or treatment outcome biomarkers foresee the course of a disorder or response to intervention, helping in designing optimal treatments for a given patient.

2.2. Biomarkers in Alzheimer's Disease

Biomarkers in the context of Alzheimer's disease, among clinical features of cognitive decline, are prominently in the limelight today. In the last 20 years, attention has been given to "biomarkers", with an increase of reports on this topic from around just ten citations from 1970 until 1990 to around one thousand publications per year in the last decade. This reflects the substantial interest in a biological definition of the disease. Levels of protein aggregates (accumulating into fibrillary tangles or extracellular plaques) have mainly been detected by means of qualitative histological assessment, which, in turn, can also be quantified through more objective image acquisition. Electrophysiology or genetic mutations in at-risk population can anticipate the incidence of the disease in certain conditions, making these also "biomarkers". Overall, biomarkers can be assessed by measuring either brain physiology metabolism, connectivity, perfusion, and atrophy or cerebrospinal fluid (CSF) protein levels. The value of biomarkers, also called "biomarker fidelity", can be addressed in neuropsychological testing. Neuropsychology is a clinical discipline focusing on the interactions between a patient's clinical condition and his neuropsychological performance; the ultimate goal of such an approach is to help diagnose the patient's illness. Thus, focusing on the neuropsychological variables can be important as it can help differentiate patients from healthy controls.

Alzheimer's disease is, by nature, a very slow decline, making diagnosis complicated, particularly in the earlier stages of the illness. A consensus of the 68th American Academy of Neurology Conference has defined biomarkers as "an objective indicator that is measured accurately and reproducibly, provides information about the formation of Alzheimer's pathology, and subsequently serves as an indicator of response to treatment." Biomarkers can be measured in biological fluids like blood or cerebrospinal fluid, as well as in imaging like Magnetic Resonance Imaging or Positron Emission Tomography. It is important to validate a method to consider an assay truly a biomarker.

Introduction

3. Importance of Early Diagnosis

While several methods are used to diagnose dementia, many have specificities close to those of AD. This promotes the development of positive and downstream diagnostic algorithms. Established AD CSF core and PET core AD biomarkers now cover all three core pathophysiologic domains of the revised NIA-AA framework. They seem eligible for their upcoming use in the diagnosis of preclinical AD as well. In summary, defining the presence of AD pathology early in the symptomatic phase at population-based level is important for different reasons. Identifying patients with AD at early stages is crucial since therapy should be initiated as soon as possible for reasons of maximal brain plasticity and plasticity of other organ systems which influence cognitive performance.

Dementia with Alzheimer's disease (AD) pathology is a devastating neurological disorder with a slow and insidious onset, which is burdensome for both patients and caregivers. Since it is thought that AD pathology begins 15-20 years before the onset of symptoms, the need for early and accurate diagnosis is crucial not only to reduce disease progression, symptoms, and costs but also to accurately identify the molecular signatures at an early stage of the AD pathological cascade, when potential disease-modifying therapies can be more effective. The burden of dementia and particularly of AD is expected to continue to increase over the years and to put a substantial pressure on healthcare systems. Besides its effect on public policy, the increase in dementia prevalence will also put significant stress on informal carers who will be faced with the task of providing care for a longer time and who will need to acquire relevant information to be better equipped for this task. In this scenario, the development of prevention strategies and of accurate and fast diagnostic means is imperative.

4. Current Diagnostic Methods

The holy grail in AD diagnosis is a diagnostic test that is able to accurately and reliably stratify people with AD and mild cognitive impairment onto a suitable treatment arm in clinical trials and thus to establish whether and how a potential treatment is working. As a result, there has been much focus on the identification of biomarkers that may be able to perform this key function. Due to the blood-brain barrier, these biomarkers are not as readily detectable in blood and cerebrospinal fluid when compared with the brain. Recent technological advances have enabled the implementation of large-scale protein quantifications within the blood across multiple research laboratories and projects.

Overall, imaging technologies can enable the relative amount of amyloid and tau in the brain to be calculated compared to age-matched healthy controls or within the same individual as a measure of suitable treatment options with disease-modifying drugs and/or a marker of disease risk. Currently, cognitive testing is time-consuming and requires an expert assessment and interpretation of patient responses.

Diagnosing dementia can be an exhaustive process and is currently predominantly based on cognitive testing, named the gold standard of dementia diagnosis. Imaging techniques have been developed and are becoming more commonly used in research settings to visually identify amyloid plaques, tau tangles, and to quantitatively measure the size and activity of brain structures affected by AD. In addition, it is thought that these technologies could potentially assist in the diagnosis of AD and mild cognitive impairment caused by AD, especially in those with a younger age of onset.

Alzheimer's Disease (AD) currently has no cure, and a definitive diagnosis can typically be made only after death, with the confirmation of amyloid beta plaques and tau tangles in the brain. The average life expectancy post-diagnosis is estimated to be around seven years for people who are already experiencing symptoms. So, the earlier a diagnosis can be made, the better the range of interventions that could help to slow or halt the progression of dementia.

Current Diagnostic Methods for Alzheimer's Disease

4.1. Cognitive Testing

Regarding cognition tests, they should provide continuous scores to inform about the brain area integrity and not only a categorical classification. This is an advantage to produce more policy evidence about the "prosecution bias" (more than clinical suspicion) of the subjects who actively collaborate in the scientific trials of dementia in general. It is "gene-based biomarker-based classification" or "bio fluid-based level of abnormal Aβ" that gives us a probability of a euthymic cognitively normal "transitory isolated subjective cognitive disorders (with profound impairment in the register capacity) at clinical (not only neuro histo-pathology) bases of non-amnestic MCI and of typical Alzheimer's disease (with typical amnestic MCI).

Biomarkers may someday supplement or enhance some current procedures for diagnosing Alzheimer's disease. Therefore, some procedures for degenerative dementias do not deserve to be applied in cognitively normal people without preventive disease-modifying treatment. The procedures include cognition testing. More than a method to measure temporal cognitive disorders, they are distinct methods that reveal distinct cognitive features preferentially amplified according to the brain regions where they are used as prior methods of usual clinical history.

4.2. Imaging Techniques

Imaging techniques such as computed tomography (CT) and magnetic resonance imaging (MRI) were first adapted to brain imaging to reveal hallmark pathologies such as atrophy or, in rare cases, hemorrhaging. CT exposed subjects to unnecessarily high dosages of ionizing radiation that structurally deteriorated the brains of elderly individuals at risk of AD. An increased atrophy in AD brains is observed in brain CT images in which the lateral ventricles appear significantly enlarged compared to age-matched healthy individuals; in this transversal plane of the images, it will then suggest correlations between a larger ventricle size and worse remembered words in delayed free recall. The simultaneously developed MRI technique detects the same pattern of atrophy in the temporal lobe with an equally high sensitivity and specificity, while providing the same results in VBM studies. In the 2000s, interstitial structural-functional technologies and the next generation, unbiased VBM techniques on larger datasets were used to identify atrophy patterns in state-of-the-art MRI processing, as well as the volume of particular regions of interest.

4.2.2. CT and MRI in use since the 80s.

Seventy-nine cases of confirmed AD and control subjects were included in this study. The subjects were examined to create an energy landscape of the hippocampal data space using the Fisher information. Results suggest that changes in the 3D architecture of a Fisher energy landscape might be globally altered and computationally sampled above the statistically significant level (p < 0.001) by AD. Moreover, the present simulation suggests that the electroencephalography data measured on the scalp can convolve the hippocampal edema in four different phases. When computing the C value for the low resolution and for the direct experimental diagnostic FP and FN results, the convolution between the high and low resolution data intensifies, improving the first-order process. The effect of the inserts can result in a SWR (slowing wave ratio), which compared with the normal patients, generates an improved path concerning the PH by compensating for the WLD effect of the zip inserter (p < 0.0002) but does not reach the 3.68 necessary level measured in AUC for diagnostic criteria (p < 0.3969).

4.2.1. Electroencephalogram may detect hippocampal edema.

5. Challenges in Alzheimer's Diagnosis

Although the vast majority of cases are the result of amyloid and tau proteins, some are not, making the diagnosis of someone with FTD complex. Patients with FTD and other diseases are often instead diagnosed with progressive supranuclear palsy or corticobasal degeneration. Although they are unique autopsy-confirmed diseases, these clinical diagnoses include individuals with Alzheimer's disease and even amyotrophic lateral sclerosis. Both diseases do seem to be caused by the accumulation of proteins in cells throughout the brain. Brains of patients with AD contain substantial quantities of two types of protein. The first is amyloid deposits that are found in the space between neurons, suppressing brain function and metabolism. The second protein that is found in AD is tau - a protein that is found within neurons performing several cellular functions including microtubule stabilization. When phosphorylated, large quantities of these proteins stop working properly and clump in twisted tangles.

Alzheimer's disease presents many of the same challenges that FTD does. A definitive diagnosis is often impossible until decades after the first symptoms arise, and even then, a brain biopsy after death is the only way to guarantee clinical diagnoses. The main diagnosis in living individuals is done by mental status examinations, neuropsychological evaluations, and medical histories. However, these tools are not perfect - minority patients present with atypical symptoms, like depression and vertigo, that make dementia seem like a less likely cause. This makes the average time to an AD diagnosis for Black and non-Black patients longer than it is for white patients.

6. Role of Biomarkers in Alzheimer's Diagnosis

4. The preferred method of neuroimaging is a scintigraphy-based system to image cerebral Aβ amyloid deposition using "Pittsburgh compound B (PiB)" or related compounds ("florbetapir," "flutemetamol," or "florbetaben"). Aβ also can be visualized by PET imaging.

3. The presence of 42-amino acid amyloid β peptides, a proteolyzed product of intra-axonal intramembranous cleavage of APP mainly by enzymes referred to as γ-secretases.

2. Amyloid Precursor Protein (APP), Nonamyloid Beta Precursor Protein (N-APP), and soluble APPβ are produced by extracellular β-secretase and α-β secretase site processing.

1. Neurofilament light chains, Tau protein, and phosphorylated Tau (P-Tau), specific proteins present in cerebrospinal fluid that reflect the accumulation of intraneuronal neurofibrillary tangle assemblies of hyperphosphorylated Tau.

Biomarkers are required not only for early diagnosis but also for monitoring therapeutic efficiency and disease progression. In recent decades, advances in molecular biology methods have resulted in the identification of several putative biomarkers for AD, among which neuroimaging and biochemical markers have gained the most attention. These biomarkers have so far been able to provide the maximum accuracy in the diagnosis of the disease. The recommended biomarkers are also included in the A-T-N classification system produced by the NIA-AA, which used a mix of 4.1 accumulated markers:

6.1. How Biomarkers Are Used

In healthy late-life individuals with no cognitive impairment, the rate of change of all three indices may be so slow as to be imperceptible at the tail end of potential lifespan, but overall the differing trajectories have led to the suggestion of reflecting "preclinical," "prodromal," and "dementia" time periods that can be conceptualized in psychological mechanisms and therapeutic interventions. Identifying high risk individuals within populations even without a cognitive concern is the main use of AD biomarkers at this time, though they have broad use in ruling out Alzheimer's – less than 1% of individuals without a biomarker or a significant genetic history will develop dementia related to $A\beta$.

The landscape of biomarkers has also expanded over the last 50 years, but for AD the specific overlap between AD dementia pathology and that of Parkinson disease (PD) has made these techniques particularly important. The physiological role of biomarkers is to extract characteristic information to help clinicians distinguish between different stages of a disease. The accumulation of beta amyloid ($A\beta$) is the earliest developed marker, and can be reliably seen 10-20 years before the earliest stages of significant memory loss. Tau, a second AD biomarker, becomes dysregulated about 5-8 years later. Both of those changes occur 1-2 decades before any cognitive loss/items on a neuropsychological test – unlike cognition, for which data suggest that change occurs on a nearly linear basis, the rise of Aβ, tau, and cognition seem to be cut with exponential time.

6.2. Types of Biomarkers Used in Diagnosis

Pathology biomarkers are primarily used in order to be able to verify the possible processes which underlie the observed clinical syndrome/neurocognitive symptoms and to be able to differentiate among specific processes. The diagnostic part thus includes the distinction of different etiology and other, potentially treatable, etiology. Further functions in clinical practice, research, and pharmaco- and physico-therapy development of both biomarker types are also discussed. A pragmatic definition of the term "biomarker" is given, too. Biomarker of associated functional deficit, then, is defined as a biological effect of the processes covering the tissue, pathology, higher cortical region, whose morphological traces are also detected by the pathology biomarkers. As a structure, it is a part of the so-called pathotopically pathological network caused by the processes mentioned above in a more cortical modality of cortical network.

In order to better understand the broad approaches to using biomarkers in the diagnosis of Alzheimer's disease, it is useful to specify their place in the diagnostic processes. From this point of view, diagnostically used biomarkers can be classified according to different criteria, below determined by the practical function and localization of the biological process addressed. The set of the biological process addressed then defines the circular and multidimensional role of diagnostic biomarkers. Guided by this character, two defining types of diagnostic biomarkers are used, namely biomarkers of pathology and those characterizing a functional deficit.

7. Advancements in Biomarker Research

Further evidence is likely to be collected in coming years about the added value of AD biomarkers and how meta-analyses may further delineate these finer characteristics. The shift to prevention will put more weight towards biomarkers with the greatest certainty of their presence in the brain prior to, during, or shortly after the initial laying down of AD pathology. Finally, involving an economic approach early on in disease, using a combination of biomarkers and predicting technology like artificial intelligence, is likely to smooth the process of intervention. What remains is the real world of clinics and in the community. It is these where constant support is needed, particularly from the community of the scientific and clinical world, to avoid the multiplication of expensive investigations without added value.

In the last decade, the concept of Alzheimer's disease (AD) biomarkers has advanced significantly. Molecular and imaging biomarkers are increasingly being included in clinical trials. Some imaging methods have even achieved a relatively clear and accepted position in programs such as those of the USA National Institute of Health or the European Union in their various clinical trial application guides. These advancements, as well as our growing understanding of AD's molecular aspects, constitute a solid foundation to understand what could potentially be used in routine clinical care for patients, from diagnosis to prognosis. Measurement of CSF amyloid and tau, plasma neurofilament light (NfL), as well as amyloid PET scan and FDG-PET remains investigational but has reached the point of possibly being used in select patients, as pointed out by a recent international working group. As hammering of these adverse findings persisted throughout the last 40 years, it now seems that biomarkers have reached a sort of benchmark of validation.

The role of biomarkers in diagnosing Alzheimer's disease

8. Clinical Applications of Biomarkers

'All' clinical applications focus on the role of biomarkers in either diagnostic decision making and/or increasing diagnostic confidence in people with SMC and MCI. Such a focus was necessary given that 'Definite' AD could only be achieved after post-mortem assessment. However, the significant need for early detection means that such a narrow application of the potential of biomarkers, particularly tau, in particular comes at a significant cost. There are currently 80 dementia subtypes and until diagnostic applications for rare dementias that incorporate different domains and temporal profiles are developed, we are essentially ignoring rare neurodementias. In addition, all proposed clinical applications of biomarkers in dementia use a binary outcome of AD vs non-AD. This makes practical sense to some extent given that treatments that would be influenced by such an outcome, such as anti-amyloid and anti-tau agents, are still being developed. However, it is also true that the utility of tau-PET in differentiating primary age related tauopathy from mild behavioural impairment has shown that a 3-way comparison could substantially increase diagnostic confidence.

This suggests that biomarkers are most clinically useful - and have the greatest ability to influence therapeutic decision making - when their information is combined with a variety of other assessments (preferences of patients with MCI, assessments of caregiver questionnaires, psychiatric history specialism diagnosis, functional MRI studies, sTREM 2, and calculation of an aggregate score). Accordingly, a composite AD diagnostic score derived from the Alzheimer's Disease Neuroimaging Initiative (ADNI) has been shown to show higher diagnostic accuracy than individual measures but would benefit from adding more variable to it. ADNI 1 patients were used to derive 11 cerebrospinal fluid (CSF)/imaging variables into an AD composite score. Combining these variables improved the prediction of an AD diagnosis more than using any of the variables on its own.

9. Ethical Considerations in Biomarker Use

Ethical commentators worldwide have argued that, while research on and the practical application of biomarkers for AD is legitimate, there must be greater public dialogue and health professional education about their benefits, limitations, and implications, to ensure those who offer or decline the tests for themselves or where they hold substitute judgment are significantly informed. In formal guidelines on the responsible conduct of biomarker-based research on mental disorders, the Global Neuroethics Summit Consensus Statement of 2018 further recommended that the generation of evidence be prioritized, and that studies report the extent to which people living with the conditions under investigation (where appropriate) have participated, might benefit from (if the test is accurate), refused or dropped out of neuroimaging research (and why), and whether/how the tests might affect their autonomy and/or the exercise of sociopolitical and economic rights. These suggestions foreground equity and the social implications of an intervention that can only be ethically justified if further research shows it is justified for wider use.

How clinicians and policy makers integrate biomarkers that are moderately predictive of Alzheimer's disease (AD) neuropathologic changes later in life into clinical practice, particularly when their only intended use is earlier AD diagnosis and prognosis, implicates a number of ethical concerns. In the public debate to date, much attention has been paid to such concerns, but the discussion has focused disproportionately on personal rather than professional responsibilities, and on the risk of self-fulfilling prophecies and chilling effects on neurology research rather than the specter of widening social inequities in access to the hope of benefits for which there is at present little or no evidence. Biomarkers for AD are not—and are not expected to become—sufficiently predictive of whether research participants will eventually develop sporadic AD to be independently medically action-guiding for any given individual. For this and other reasons, their accuracy and utility (against competitors, if they exist) is still far from clear.

10. Future Directions and Potential Impact

Ultimately, the intention of many is to prevent death to dementia-causing amyloids or at least prevent the amyloid-positive, tau positive and even possibly tuned normal-aging at the beginning of dementia rather than to detect dementias at Alzheimer's dementia, but identifying other populations out known risk factors for dementia, who also need to be preempted or managed, and 100% sensitivity of having one symptom of Alzheimer is not paramount to achieve that.

Incorporating large-scale biomarker testing into clinical care so that everyone receives either long-term follow-up as a -/- or treat/care plan as a +/- while only requiring a more expensive -/+ or +/- to get the amyloid-PET or lumbar puncture used to assess one case and the normal aging respectively.

Three major areas of future research are as follows: First, establishing the denominative cutpoints for classifying low or high tau to be used across diverse patient populations. Given that median CSF conditions will overposition the tau/I3 groups relative to the td/I3 groups and high CSF I1 need to be explored. Second, conducting studies in younger age brackets to determine whether detecting PET or CSF aβ or tau measures in a mid-adult or middle-aged population is even useful for the dementia outcome in old age. Third is exploration of what other neurological or systemic phenomena measure (e.g., autonomic dysfunction assessed by skin nerve or heart measurements or genetic traits) could improve accuracy over detecting abnormal aβ and tau proteopathy in the two most brain regions with subsequent standard radi, etc. There may also be measurements already available in the electronic health record that can improve diagnostic accuracy for Alzheimer's.

11. Conclusion

Biomarkers have the potential to improve the diagnosis of Alzheimer's disease (AD). They may help to detect those who will progress to an advanced stage of the disease at an earlier time, either by visualizing AD pathologic changes in vivo and/or indirectly detecting neurodegeneration. In conducting this review, the Amyloid Biomarker Research Working Group acknowledged that these pathologic processes can only ever be indirectly associated with underlying AD pathobiology and, at present, are not AD-specific. Whether our concept of AD will shift to being a 'biomarker'-based diagnosis in the future is not yet clear, but emerging work is beginning to shed light on both the complexity and heterogeneity of 'underlying AD pathobiology'. To date, large-scale neuropathologic evaluations of the oldest of the old have only reported that a proportion, not all, have sufficient AD pathologic changes to meet pathological criteria for AD.

This article addressed the role of biomarkers in diagnosing Alzheimer's disease (AD), with a focus on amyloid-β, total tau, and phosphorylated tau. We evaluated these biomarkers across three diagnostic algorithms: (i) those established by the National Institute on Aging and the Alzheimer's Association, (ii) the International Working Group, and (iii) the Amyloid Biomarker Research Working Group. Biomarkers performed similarly according to all three diagnostic algorithms, with potential cut-offs identified for biomarker positivity and negativity to detect the different stages of AD. Along with recent advances in unraveling the complexity and heterogeneity of AD, these core biomarkers may improve diagnostic accuracy and even revolutionize how we diagnose and monitor the disease.

The Role of Biomarkers in Disease Diagnosis and Treatment

1. Introduction to Biomarkers

Predictive biomarkers are useful for the selection of patients who are most likely to respond to a particular target therapy. Predictive markers provide information about the likelihood of response. Several diagnostic tests, perhaps in combination, may be required to provide an effective diagnosis and prediction of outcome in confirmed cases of patients with conditions such as systemic infections to be treated with antibiotics. The development of high throughput genomics and proteomic tools have revolutionised the approach towards the identification of biomarkers. Many of the high throughput technologies are limited by the quantitative sensitivity or require expensive instrumentation and reagents and exhibit low reproducibility. Typically, classifiers based on genomic, proteomic, and metabolomic data provide high sensitivity and specificity approaching 90% or higher.

Biomarkers are regarded as valuable for the diagnosis and treatment of a diverse set of diseases, including cancer, heart disease, asthma and allergy, depression, and mental illnesses. A biomarker is a tool which can be utilised to monitor the magnitude of biological variation due to a disease or a therapeutic intervention. It can be categorised into genomic, transcriptomic, proteomic, glycomic, lipidomic, cellomic, metabonomic and imaging biomarkers based on the type of molecules. Biomarkers based on their principle of operation can be classified into prognostic, predictive, diagnostic, and theranostic. The sensitivity and specificity of a particular diagnostic test often depend on the method used in its detection, sample collection, precaution taken during sample collection and sample sizes. The major benefit of the biomarker test is objective evidence of the presence of an infectious pathogen, which can be provided in a much more rapid timeframe than current culture methods.

1.1. Definition and Types of Biomarkers

There are expected changes in people with a certain ailment, such as elevated plasma creatine kinase in myocardial infarction. Furthermore, biomarkers are divided into rules and therapeutic categories. A drug response biomarker can demonstrate changes in the body's reaction that help treatment management. In many tests, approaches to specific drugs are established when the patient is identified as a promising responder or non-responder in disease diagnosis. Notably, specific medications aid in the collection of toxic produced drugs in several individuals due to the variations in the capacity of drug processing. Further observations at observations indicate the biomarkers correlated with the risk of anomalies and the aquar, such as birth, weight, frequency of anomalies corresponding to a specified dose of a given substance for in utero exposure. Biomarkers can help to reduce the occurrence of signs of certain toxic outcomes, such as lung or blistering injuries that are used in biochemical data measurements, and they have not been used in coronary or vascular interventions following a single 40.imens containing special universal cardiovascular disease demographics. Biomarkers may aid in decisions with clinical significance. For reasons such as invasive sampling to obtain proof, they have a higher predictive power than many conventional sources of evidence, e.g., clinical and geographic ecology, and human demography. When appropriate for the purpose, they predict early illnesses or the possibility of sequel. In a wide variety of clinical and community-based applications, their potential should be checked.

A biomarker refers to a measurable physical characteristic that predicts life processes and the absence or presence of disease. Moreover, biomarkers cover different measurable characteristics, including toxicants, genetic mutations, and risk estimates. A biomarker may indicate the established risk of future diseases, such as a lipid lipoprotein. They can reflect a likelihood of future diseases, such as coronary calcification (carotid intima-media total).

1.2. Importance of Biomarkers in Disease Diagnosis

For example, enzymes such as lactate dehydrogenase, which are biomarkers, particularly those that are well known (LDL), in the diagnosis as acute myocardial infarction. Inflammatory biomarkers, including C-reactive protein (CRP), serum amyloid A, and the adhesion molecules such as intercellular adhesion molecule-1 (ICAM-1) and E-selectin, have been advocated to be useful biomarkers of the mild level of acute systemic inflammatory response in order to respond to acute myocardial infarction. In addition, the enzyme troponin, which has been demonstrated to be an acute marker of myocardial infarction, is slightly higher in patients with infectious myocarditis. Markers of myocarditis include acute phase proteins, immunological markers, nitric oxide, enzymes, and acute phase proteins. Disease diagnosis may also take place through imaging using magnetic resonance imaging (MRI) as a biomarker (myocarditis).

Biomarkers are of critical importance for disease diagnosis. Disease, defined as a steady state deviation from the normal state, cannot be properly diagnosed and thus treated without the ability to make a comparison between the diseased state and a normal condition. Although diagnostic imaging techniques provide useful information for the diagnosis of diseases, blood tests have, for years, been the preferred method of disease diagnosis, and this is more accurate than many imaging techniques. Indeed, the striking showcase of the significance of blood examination is that nearly all, if not all, clinical assessments of the functions of internal organs, such as the heart, kidney, and liver, and the diagnosis of cardiovascular diseases, infectious diseases, cancer, and even serious diseases resulting from the inheritance of mutant genes, rely predominantly on blood tests.

2. Biomarkers in Neurodegenerative Diseases

Alzheimer's disease (AD), the leading cause of senile dementia, is characterized by a long presymptomatic phase, showing potential benefit for biomarker measures for early diagnosis and assessment of response to therapy. More than 10% of people aged over 80 years will develop dementia, and the development and course of the disease will progress with the aging population. AD incidence varies by country, and growing economies will face the greatest increase in dementia incidence, particularly in China, with growth from 3.8 to 10 million patients in the past decade. Approximately two-thirds of Alzheimer's patients are living in low- and middle-income countries. In other words, AD becomes one of the world's leading diseases. The common view that biomarkers can predict the conversion of mild cognitive impairment (MCI) to AD dementia and identify the different stages of cognitive decline in AD is of great significance. Biomarkers can also be used to monitor the progression of brain masses and assess the efficacy of new treatments. These biomarkers are largely divided into two categories: structural and functional imaging biomarkers and liquid biomarkers. Biomarkers can also be used to evaluate the early diagnosis in clinical trials and diffuse the rejection of AD treatments with adverse side effects. However, detection of some protein-specific peripheral biomarkers of AD, such as amyloid-β and tau, in the early stage of AD is likely to have a positive and important role in the prediction of AD.

There is growing evidence that many neurodegenerative diseases are accompanied by specific fluid and imaging biomarker changes, which are closely associated with pathological accumulation of various proteins. Among the most common protein aggregation diseases are Alzheimer's disease (AD), which is associated with the accumulation of hyperphosphorylated tau protein; Parkinson's disease, which is associated with the accumulation of α-synuclein protein; and transthyretin-associated amyloidosis (ATTR), which is associated with the accumulation of transthyretin and its variants. Among other proteins, Creutzfeldt-Jakob disease is associated with the accumulation of prion proteins; Huntington's disease with the accumulation of huntingtin; and frontotemporal dementias and amyotrophic lateral sclerosis with the accumulation of FUS, TDP-43, and many others.

2.1. Alzheimer's Disease Biomarkers

Amyloid beta (Aβ) and/or tau are integral to the selection of patients for clinical studies. Tau PET ligands discriminate AD dementia from controls (both amyloid positive and negative), aMCI, FTD, corticobasal degeneration, and progressive supranuclear palsy. It has been noted that while the slope from baseline of 2-3 months dual time point scans is correlated with cognitive performance in ADNI subjects, it did not show as strong associations as the 3-year scan in detecting cognitive decline. In addition, sTREM2 in plasma is also increased and correlates with $pRO2$, pointing to a potential increase in peripheral immune myeloid response as a measure inversely proportional to the immune response in the brain. These biomarkers also hold potential as early indicators of tissue damage (both trials and research) and have shown the capacity to predict future cSVD. Reduced pNfL has also been demonstrated post-acute sport-related concussion as early as 7 days.

Many of their research on neurodegenerative diseases focuses on Alzheimer's disease. Of these studies, many focus on research on Alzheimer's disease. One additional focus is the development of biomarkers such as neurofilament light chain. Research in this area is not exclusive to human patients and has particularly focused on establishing baseline values and determining whether some mammals are more relevant for translation between humans and mice. These biomarkers have long been used as tools for disease diagnosis and monitoring;

quantification in the cerebrospinal fluid (CSF) and blood has proven capable of discriminating between different dementias and MCI and is associated with dementia staging.

2.2. Parkinson's Disease Biomarkers

In the last ten years, potential biomarkers suitable for being detected in a body fluid blood have been exploited to some extent. For early diagnosis, principally at the prodromal stage, a biomarker would ideally detect an ongoing process that is present at the early stage of the disease in the range of, for instance, accumulating α-synuclein or neuroinflammation or neurodegeneration. In the early years, after the Disease Time, this pathophysiologic process should still maintain relevance. For the late stages of Parkinson's disease, a "biomarker for the disease" relates more to the growing evidence of disease through traditional lumbar puncture or blood biomarkers, mainly to exclude other pathologies from a similar clinical picture. Of note, neuroinflammatory processes appear to be disconnected from disease progression as measured in longitudinal CSF studies in early and moderate stages of PD. Thus, we restrict this section to the very few, to date generally accepted, blood biomarkers in PD and PD prodromal stages.

The continuous turnover of neurons is a huge challenge, as it is like fixing an airplane while it is flying. Neurons affected in Parkinson's disease rely on the few and selective markers that can be quantified in autopsied tissues ex vivo or via brain imaging in vivo. Relatively selective dopaminergic neurons can seriously affect behavior via functional magnetic brain imaging. Nonetheless, it is difficult to identify quantifiable biomarkers within the brain that could be measured noninvasively in the blood resulting in a diagnosis based mainly on the patient's history and clinical evaluation. Therefore, relevant generally accepted biomarkers for early diagnosis, especially at the prodromal stage (as an early indicator of the disease), have not been fully established so far. Many important genetic and environmental factors have been introduced that lower the threshold for Parkinson's disease, but stratification of the risk for disease of any individual is not based on biomarkers. Stratification into different subtypes of Parkinson's disease in need of different treatments or as a marker of successful treatment strategy (biomarker of treatment effect) or of success in developing novel therapy (biomarker of the intended effect) is equally not based on the biomarkers for the vast majority of cases of Parkinson's disease.

3. Methods of Biomarker Detection

Many different imaging techniques can be leveraged for non-invasive measurement of these molecules and provide the additional advantage of looking at molecules in the spatial context of the body. Techniques include magnetic resonance imaging (MRI), positron emission tomography (PET), magnetic resonance spectroscopy (MRS), and others such as molecular imaging techniques and X-ray and optical imaging which are beginning to be used more commonly. The advantage of molecular imaging techniques is that they can image more than just proteins, such as genes, receptors, enzymes, and more. MRI of neurodegenerative diseases, for example, uses structural measurements of brain volume by the T1 sequence combined with the spatial resolution and contrast of the T2 sequence to help predict incidence of mild cognitive impairment for clinical trials in Alzheimer's disease. Mass spectrometry (LC-MS/MS) is commonly used in the diagnosis of cancers. Temporal sequence of genetic changes in cells during carcinogenesis explains why cancers are difficult to detect at early stages. Exome sequencing has been shown to be a useful tool for screening therapies of pancreatic cancer, where individuals with mismatch repair gene mutations had significantly better prognosis.

Laboratory methods include enzyme-linked immunosorbent assays (ELISAs), radioimmunoassays (RIAs), Western blots, and others. Though ELISAs are most commonly used, there are challenges with reproducibility and robustness that can lead to issues with translation to clinical medicine. The detection means (antibodies) and manner of usage (detection of direct protein concentration) make these difficult to advance to early diagnosis, though they are useful for understanding disease progression as a whole.

3.1. Laboratory Techniques

Each method has been improved with many technical improvements in the last 20 years, and these improvements continue to be made. Electronic microscopes are now used instead of old ones based on video digitizing, permitting magnifications up to 150,000 without altering the quality. A single word can be associated with this laboratory technique: Automation. Automations now permit different markers to be detected in the same analysis without any human intervention. The use of alternately vacuum purging and washing to have a sample devoid of red and white blood cells, with oligonucleotide probes fixed in situ, was described in 1993. A polymerase chain reaction (PCR)-based amplification of complementary c-DNA, in situ detection, and revelation by a classical substrate was used to identify a specific gene for the first time in 1997 and improved to be automated in 1999 using FV-Leiden in a 23-factor multiphasic analysis. This technique measured, beside the FV-1691-G and A factors, the FV-Leiden presence and severity, the VKORC-1 most frequent mutations, prothrombin 20210 A factor, H-FABP, and cTnI in the same analysis. LC-ESI-tandem mass spectroscopy enables us to show both creatinine and cystatin C proteins, which were used for GFR calculations. Detection of rRNA mutations has to move to this technology to be used in large placebo-controlled studies.

The first thing that will be needed is a sample prepared in the right way. The samples should be prepared for the method chosen. To use blood, urine, saliva, etc., a patient must agree and have his or her samples taken. The laboratory has to know when the collection happened because specific and non-specific changes can happen over time in the samples, which can affect the results. Many standardized methods exist to keep the samples in the best conditions until the day of the test.

Research in a laboratory setting allows for the accurate and controlled detection of biomarkers in samples. As such, scientists use laboratory techniques to identify and analyze the biomarkers in any given sample. There are a variety of different techniques that can be adapted to fit a range of needs, each with their own advantages and disadvantages. The laboratory technique chosen will have a significant impact on the study's success, but some steps have to be performed in advance of any subject.

3.2. Imaging Techniques

Imaging techniques fall into three main groups: X-ray or computed tomography (CT) imaging, magnetic resonance imaging (MRI), and positron emission tomography (PET). Of these, CT, MRI, and PET are similar in that they all use radioactive isotopes/molecules to either enhance the signal or have a radioactive signature themselves and show up in the final image. For example, in MRI and CT, the presence of a metal surface or ion is used to enhance the signal, whereas PET utilizes the principle that diseased cells or tumors have different glucose metabolisms compared to healthy tissue, which incorporates slightly radioactive glucose in a process called "fluorodeoxyglucose positron emission tomography" (FDG-PET). The actual image produced will depend on the radiotracer used as the binding partner (or ligand) which will concentrate the image on a certain part of the body, which then is shown more clearly and distinctly from the rest. For example, in new anti-cancer drug research, the new drug can be radiolabeled and its distribution and target organ examined. In disease progression, where the ischemic tissue is too small to be seen even with these advanced imaging systems, one tracer ion, gadolinium, can cause contrast enhancement to the affected region allowing physicists to define where there is still or lies in regions of ischemia (a lack of circulation), and these regions become dark in NMRI (nuclear magnetic resonance imaging).

As well as analyzing biopsy specimens in the laboratory, there are also systems for detecting biomarker proteins in the body, specifically imaging techniques. These are useful for not only visualizing the biomarker itself but also observing its distribution in the body and whether its expression is local or systemic. Moreover, paired with radiolabeled markers and tracers, these techniques are capable of distinguishing the whole range of diseases studied in this thesis.

4. Biomarkers in Precision Medicine

Precision medicine is not a synonym for the generation of more subpopulations within a disease, but to employ biomarkers to discover how to treat patients nowadays or in targeting the treatment for individual patients. Based on this biological stratification of a population, a method that uses research evidence to try to work out which treatment is likely to be most effective and best for the patient has been developed. In brief, two kinds of population stratification have been identified: biological stratification predetermine the characteristics of people most likely to get a disease or have a worse prognosis, i.e., predictors of an event, while biological stratification post-prescribe which drug or other intervention is more likely to be effective for an individual, i.e., surrogate or marker-outcome relationship. The presence or absence of these molecular markers will/can be used to decide whether a patient should or should not be given treatment, taking current therapies and risk of side effects into account. This will also demonstrate the precise nature of 'mechanisms-based' treatment axis or personalized medicine. In most clinical practice, the terms 'stratified medicine' and 'personalized medicine' are used interchangeably.

Clinical conduct has traditionally had a 'one-size-fits-all' policy towards disease diagnosis and treatment, ignoring the substantial heterogeneity within a population. Precision medicine is a medical paradigm that takes individual patient variability into account: suitable intervention depends on patient characteristics, such as lifestyle, environment, and genetic predispositions. Disease biomarkers have been identified as critical to the success of precision medicine agendas. This part of the review will examine the role of biomarkers in precision medicine diagnosis and/or prognosis.

The role of biomarkers in precision medicine

4.1. Personalized Treatment Strategies

All these strategies essentially rely on using surrogate disease endpoints to try to counterbalance the suboptimal potentials of observer-based, episodic and not organ-specific outcome measures to assess and follow the natural history of patients. Monitoring disease biomarkers as well as aging or frailty indices can guide treatment in individual subjects much earlier than the onset of complications or endpoints that require invasive monitoring, as those are the gold standard, because their association with outcome is kept along the process of revision of clinical guidelines and treatment indications. In addition, the use of endotype identification to characterize the disease in a patient or a patient subgroup does not preclude the combined use of individualized strategies that have been selected according to the concomitant conditions of the patient, such as multimorbidity, fragility, age, individual susceptibility to drug side effects, and comorbidities.

Monitoring disease biomarkers to guide treatment

The lack of success in non-personalized treatment of a number of diseases clearly underscores the need to identify subgroups of patients who derive beneficial effects from specific interventions. The best justification for using biomarkers, and probably the ultimate goal for precision medicine, is to tailor therapy to the characteristics of the individual patient. As a first step in the definition of personalization, a number of different strategies can be identified, some of which are not really disease-tailored but rather patient-tailored. Clearly, using gender as a selection criterion to treat with a drug active in both genders only at a higher individual susceptibility is not employing a disease-based personalized strategy; most disease-based individualized treatments ultimately use patient characteristics that are unrelated to the disease, such as liver function, weight, polymorphisms in enzymes active in drug metabolisms, etc.

Lack of success in non-personalized treatment

5. Challenges and Future Directions in Biomarker Research

At present, the quality, format, and standardization of the associated documentation (which are necessary for the EBM methodology to be performed) are far from ideal. Despite certain initiatives towards standardization of data, there are currently few databases profiled and focused specifically on the qualitative and quantitative meta-analysis of differential diagnosis and/or prognosis, let alone a database aligned towards the comparison of tests.

Given its nascent nature, we are now entering a second phase of development in the use of biomarker and clinical data for diagnosis, prognosis, and medicine. The high technology and data availability in this latter wave are set to overwhelm the nation's healthcare system, especially in the primary care sector, where the majority of 'gatekeeping' diagnostic, screening, assessment, investigative, and monitoring decisions are made. These methods will need adaptation and re-validation using more flexible and intelligent formats to bring us back full circle to bedside and epidemiological research involving biomarkers and the development of diagnostic and prognostic tests.

First and foremost, any studies involving biomarkers raise complex ethical issues. From an academic or research point of view, it is not expedient to collect genetic information if it is not immediately useful for the patient. In clinical studies, accordingly, any risk/benefit assessment clearly indicates that practicably useful tests should replace less reliable or more invasive ones. For studies of the performance of a 'standalone' diagnostic test in its target population, such arguments may hold even more strongly. Our successor would consider the evidence available in association studies in coming to a decision about allocating resources.

Biomarker research has advanced rapidly over the past two decades and will continue to have an immense impact on healthcare and disease management. However, as with any area emerging from its 'first wave' of expansion, the field is also facing numerous challenges that need to be addressed to accelerate further development.

4. Challenges and Future Directions

5.1. Ethical Considerations

The pros and cons of discussing issues relating to biomarkers based approaches require two new ethical concerns: (i) RTC can generate concerns as to the position of healthy patients and (ii) as to information and confidentiality policies. In the predominant approach, particular attention is paid to the interest of the individual since the individual body, like the person's thoughts and preferences, is considered sacred. If a potential harm is to be avoided, it would seem that special considerations apply in the assessment of the benefits and harms of RTD. Finally, there is a question of control over all-cause characteristics. General predictive genetic markers that indicate a broad range of disorders may be regarded as "products." Cancer is not a disease in general, just like cancer treatment cannot be applied but instead a wide array of alternative cancer treatments. On the other hand, there has been no discussion on the use of socially based markers that may reveal health information about individuals with quarter characteristics.

Developing biomarkers requires close involvement with medical specialists and policy makers in the sense that people, technological tools, and a vast amount of data need to work together in order for a biomarker to be declared clinically valid and ready for use. Because of the complexity of using, linking, interpreting, and turning to benefit the network of interactions for this set of stakeholders, the discussion of such long-term outcomes takes secondary consideration. Yet, the scientific community and the commercial parties involved are to be appreciated for driving the research on biomarkers. At the core of medical and social implications is the possibility of identifying one's consequences and the interventions that would be applied thanks to that information. Clinicians and society at large need discussion to be informed in their decision making. The use of biomarkers has been questioned for both moral and societal reasons, and some of the points raised here have been raised with respect to genetic technologies.

5.2. Technological Advancements

Evidently, the rapid advancements of technology can potentially revolutionize the implementation of personalized medicines in clinics. Furthermore, the biodegradable technology and the use of the new technologies could, in the future, assist the constant monitoring of patients, the toxins in a patient's body and assist the tracking of biomarkers automatically. The need for blood samples to be drawn on a routine basis to monitor the inflammatory activity of the bowel, following an IBD patient has been removed. While pharma has a lot to learn, if they are looking at these new developments of personalized medicines. In such cases, they should be focusing on the drugs to create the technology, diagnostics, surgery, as well as the comprehensive patient care that is required, and not just focusing on a pill. For disease diagnoses and progression there have been a number of methods used, including a simple health check performed by a professional to blood and urine samples, x-rays, biopsies and scans. All methods used will take into consideration a complete picture of your health, symptoms and results of your clinical examination.

Magalhães found "high-quality research has moved the biomarker bases, and this has improved the prospects for these potentially beneficial intervention strategies to help millions of patients presenting with sepsis." Be it through blood tests, MRIs, or the tracking of assisted everyday motions and activities, it is increasingly accessible to modern medicine and research. Continued advances could be used in blood tests as the future method in the early identification of a stroke, abnormal proteins in the brain as a definitive diagnosis for Alzheimer's. With regards to mental health, we can see in the case of an EEG, known as electroencephalography. This examines electrical activity in the brain is an innovative approach to diagnosing and treating psychiatric disorders such as mood disorders and anxiety. Complete with FDA clearance, this tool has managed to decode brainwaves, potentially identifying adolescents and adults, who are at higher risk than normal of suicidal tendencies based on "prefrontal theta cord synchronization".

The first generation significantly increased our understanding of biomarker roles and functions. This is not only beneficial for diagnosis, but appears to be even more useful for therapy monitoring and patient management. However, ethical considerations are of extreme importance and, as such, patient care is the priority over and above any financial motives. Part of personalized medicine, also known as precision medicine and systemic treatment, is the use of adjuvant therapies to alter our immune pathology. This process profiles the testing for biomarkers to ensure that we are administering the correct medication in a timely manner. However, the window of opportunity is closing somewhat, with the rapid advancement of technology and science due to the fact that more and more medical conditions having several treatment types and options. This will ultimately lead to increased complexities for cancer treatment primarily, which is not only to deal with cancer itself but also must coincide with the damaging, severe, and often life-threatening toxicities that treatments such as radiation and chemotherapy may succumb to.